Eczema And The Food We Eat

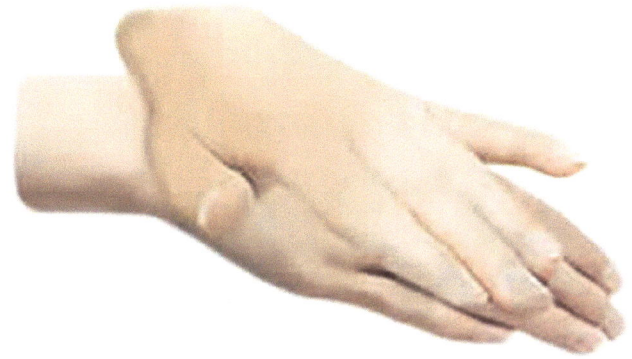

Cure Your Eczema The Natural Way With Delicious 100% All Natural Homeopathic Whole Grain Herbal Salads

Donald Ridgeway
Sacramento, California

This Book Is Dedicated To All People Suffering From Eczema And Chronic Skin Disorders.

Get relief the natural way not only for skin problems related to Eczema. These All Natural Herbal Salads also help relieve skin problems related to Chilblains, Erysipelas, Fistulas, Herpes, Psoriasis, Scabies, Scrofula sores, Sciatica, Scurf, Acne and more.

Eczema And The Food We Eat

Published by   RCMG-Publishing
Copyright © 2011   RCMG-Publishing
Cover Copyright © 2011   RCMG-Publishing

Title ID: *Eczema And The Food We Eat*

10 9 8 7 6 5 4 3

First Edition first printing: May 2014

Printed in the United States Of America

Contents

Eczema And The Food We Eat
All Natural Grain Diet

Supplementary Omaga-3 Homeopathic Herbal Salads to help cure
Eczema and other skin related problems

Introduction

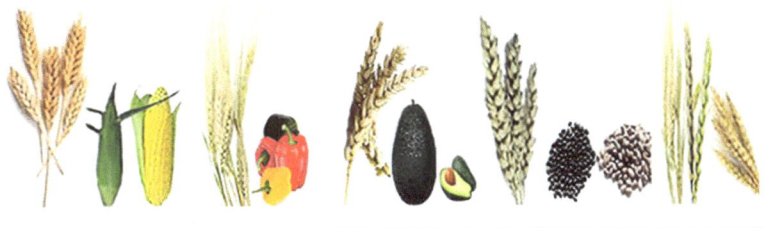

You know the saying, YOU ARE WHAT YOU EAT, and the same holds true for the treatment of your Eczema dermatitis and other skin problems. In other words, it is important to take in consideration the foods that we consume in order to help control the problem. Below are some things that you should consider to help you with your eczema problem. Keep an eye out for the types of *foods* that causes your *eczema* to flare-up. Some *foods* such as shell fish, nuts and others can be allergic to some people… Raw foods like fruits, vegetables, and sprouts are known to have a marked effect on the B-cells function. These cells are the lymphocytes which play a big role in the humoral immune response, functioning mainly to make antibodies fight against antigens. So in short, these raw foods boost the production of lymphocytes in order to enhance the body's resistance to ill-health. By taking in raw foods, the body is supplied with good quantities of vitamins A, C, E, B, and zinc. This then will result in a powerful immune system, protecting the body from diseases like eczema and maintaining smooth and healthier skin. But let's first be clear on one thing.

But before I go any further, I would like to say that, I am not a doctor. But I have studied and worked with holistic medicines for many years, I hardly ever go to the doctor and have for the last 30 years or so mixed my won preparation for whatever ails me and my family.

Introduction

Herbalism, the knowledge and study of herbs may not be a term in your active vocabulary but a definite reality in your life. The mustard on your table and many of the other spices on your kitchen shelf comes from herbs. Most of the vegetables in your salad are herbs.

So what is a HERB?

The term herb is often applied more generally to any plant part or all of which has been used for such purposes as medical treatments, nutritional value, food seasoning, coloring or dying of other substances. Historically the most important uses for herbs were medical. Folk medicine from the early days until the twentieth century was mainly prepared at home, in fact folk medicine is the household use of simple herbal remedies, based on word of mouth tradition that probably stretches in an unbroken line of Prehistoric times. Prehistoric man used plants to treat physical complaints, he also used them for food and shelter long before written history began. He undoubtedly learned by instinct and by generations of trial and error that certain plants could be used for treating illnesses and disease. The ancient Greeks and Romans valued plants for their various uses for medicine, symbols and magic charms, for food seasoning, cosmetics, dyes etc., but the uses of plants for medicine and other purposes changed very little during the middle ages. The early Christian churches discouraged the formal practice of medicine preferring faith healing, but many Greek and Roman writings of medicines and other subjects were preserved by diligent hand copying of manuscripts in monasteries. The monasteries thus tended to become local centers for medical knowledge and their herbal gardens provided the raw materials for several treatments for common disorders. At the same time folk medicine in the home and villages continued uninterrupted supporting numerous travelling and settled herbalist.

During that time a herb that had a reputation for healing might fine itself prescribed by a peasant grand mother, sold by a wondering herbalist, charmed as an ingredient for a magic potion or amulet by a wise woman. Or a quark compounded into a complex and often vile mixture to be dispensed by a physician in the hope that it would drive out whatever possessed the patient. The importance of herbs for the centuries following the Middle Ages is indicated by hundreds of herbal publication after the invention of printing in the 15th century. The basic assumption behind natural healing is that man is part of a continuum of being. Since he is a living being physical and mental condition is linked especially to properties and influences of natural organic substances. Many of these in various quantities are necessary for life itself, others are valuable if not essential for maintaining the body at it's optimum state of health. The trend in the cosmetic industry for instance is headed more and more toward natural cosmetics made from natural plant and animal substances with few or no chemical additives. These cosmetics are more beneficial for your skin than most other chemical preparations which are almost totally, composed of chemical ingredients. Almost all cosmetic companies, especially the big ones now days offer more natural items, but the best selection of natural cosmetics can generally be found in health food stores, especially herbs that help control acne, eczema and other types of skin disorders. All commercial natural cosmetics tend to be expensive-fortunately you can make many natural beauty preparations yourself at a much lower cost. Many of these are based on home herbal treatment receipts that have been used successfully for centuries. Most of these herbs are used medically to treat skin disorders and they have also been found to be beneficial to the skin for cosmetic purposes and healing.

Allergies

Now you might ask-how did I get a Food Allergy? Often when a child is allergic, there are family members with allergies or a tendency for allergies to be passed on. Others develop allergies with no apparent genetic background. Treatment is generally one of three approaches: largely it involves **avoidance** of the allergen whenever possible, **treatment and management** of symptoms, or **auto-immune therapy, injections** of extracts of the allergen to try and de-sensitise the individual. Therefore, when choosing a diet for your eczema, there are several factors that you need to consider in order to reduce flare ups, all the while ensuring that you get the nutrients that you need to be a healthy and thriving individual. So, in your quest to cure your illness you should consider four things:

- Foods Commonly Known To Trigger Eczema
- Determining What Foods Cause Your Flare-Ups
- Add Food Substitutes To Ensure Proper Nutrition
- Incorporating Foods That Aid In Eczema Relief

Logically, the first step in choosing a diet to help cure your eczema involves getting to know the common foods that have been proven to trigger such aggravating and often painful flare ups. As a norm the most commonly known foods that trigger eczema flare-ups include the following:

- Eggs
- Dairy
- Wheat
- Gluten
- Nuts
- Citrus Fruits
- Soy
- Tomatoes
- Chocolate
- Shell Fish

Here are some substitute foods that you can use in place of the one's which are causing your eczema to flare up...

- Soybean varieties - soy is a great substitute for dairy.
- Spelt & Rye - a great substitute for wheat.
- Beans are a great substitute for eggs.
- Kiwi's are a great substitute for citrus.
- Salmon - a great addition to the diet of the eczema sufferer, provides a good source of EFA's
- Pumpkin seeds are a great addition to the eczema sufferers diet.
- Sunflower seeds- perfect for the eczema sufferers diet.
- Chickpeas - is another great addition to an eczema sufferers diet.

Now we are going to take a closer look at the foods and supplements that can help turn your eczema around, and these will be presented in the form of *All Natural Homeopathic Herbal Salads.* Once you know what foods are potential eczema triggers, you can transition to the next step....

Part I

Your 100% All Natural Homeopathic Grain Diet

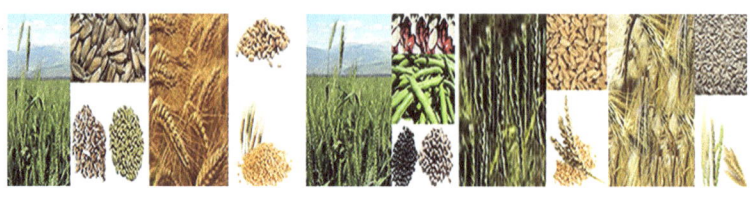

You can you depend 100% on an improved all natural grain diet as the only remedy for reversing eczema. Food allergies are an autoimmune response caused by the body "misreading" a food protein as an enemy or toxic substance. You know what they say, YOU ARE WHAT YOU EAT... And the treatment of your Eczema dermatitis skin problems should be #1 one your list. In other words, it is important to take in consideration the foods that one consumes in order to help control the problem.

I think that most of us know what skin disorders such as acne and eczema are and the particular effects that they have on the individual and family members. There are many different types of skin disorders and eczema for instance affects millions of people world wide. I have personally witnessed with my own eyes the effects that almost all types of eczema has on the body and mind. Nummular eczematous dermatitis is one of them. Of course you know that there exits all kinds of information about acne, eczema and other skin disorders and it would be in my case a bit redundant to try and add any new information or something that you probably already know about. The skin problems that many people have on their body, hands and feet usually starts when they are in adolescence or after contact with irritants. And like an ugly shadow, it follows them around and about for years which also causes lot's of pain and embarrassment.

With nearly 30 million people affected with eczema in the United States alone, its no wonder that eczema is the #1 reason people visit the dermatologist. Powerful treatments are being developed as a result of new research that has identified the genes responsible for eczema. And the trend in the cosmetic industry for instance is headed more and more toward natural.

Cure your Eczema the all natural Way. This book is a comprehensive guide to gentle, safe and effective treatment for Eczema chronic and irritating skin. Just remember, you should always use 100% All Natural whole foods and not man-made supplements.

Support - foods digestion and assimilation through the use of enzyme and probiotics supplements.
Nourish - consuming nutrient rich foods such as wheat grass, bee pollen, blue green algae etc.
Repair - protect your body through the use of whole food antioxidant supplements such as wheat sprouts, red algae, wheat grass and against free radical damage. The 100% All **Grain Natural Diet**, protecting the skin from **Free Radical Damage**, and natural **Healing Through Detoxification**-this model to finding nutritional treatment for eczema, which is the same as the Nutritional Medical Model, and the same model which my brother used to cure his Eczema irritated skin is one of the best solutions on the market. I am 100% sure that with this book and the different amazingly nutritional and good tasting receipts for my all natural

grain eczema curing salads will help accelerate the healing process of many forms of eczema and other skin conditions. Below are some foods that you should consider trying to help cure your eczema problems.

Avocado:

Avocado will help to eliminate your eczema if included in your diet. Avocado carrier oil is quite beneficial in treating skin diseases, it is extremely beneficial in treating skin disorders such as eczema and Psoriasis. Skin problems, especially eczema and psoriasis, respond to its high content of vitamins A and E. Eat lots of avocados and other foods high in EFAs (essential fatty acids) not only will your eczema be under control you will feel great all the time.

Barley:

BARLEY grass may be used to alleviate eczema. The high chlorophyll content in BARLEY grass gives it strong cleansing properties and helps to get rid of toxins in the body. Many people are allergic to Buckwheat, and if you are, try an alternative grain for the salads mentioned below. BARLEY Grass (12 grams of BARLEY Grass powder administered in 3 x 4 gram dosages per day) may alleviate eczema in up to 75% in some people.

Beans:

Bean pods are effective in lowering blood sugar levels in the body. Prolonged use of a bean decoction is recommended for difficult cases of acne. You can also apply it directly to the skin for moist eczema eruptions.

Buckwheat whole grains:

Buckwheat is the seed of the herbaceous plant Fagopyrum

esculentum Moench and has been used as a homeopathic medicine in cases of severe itching and eczema skin disorders. Buckwheat tea is used to cure circulatory problems. It is used in the treatment of chilblain, retinitis, eczema and liver disorders.

Corn:

Even though some people have an intolerance to corn, others don't. Corn is a common food that may act as a trigger to your eczema eruptions. Eating organic corn may help to get rid of this problem, and it has helped control eczema in many cases. If you are allergic to corn try substituting it with chick peas.

Millet:

Millet used in combinations with other foods helps cure Atopic eczematous dermatitis which is one of the most common forms of eczema. Millet is far removed from the family of grains to which wheat belongs to. A gluten free diet is often very beneficial in treating eczema and psoriasis. Add brown rice and Millet to your diet and be sure to include plenty of fibber. The green leaves of finger Millet are valuable for treating chronic eczema. The fresh juice of these leaves should be applied over the affected area in the treatment.

Natural rice:

Eating plenty of legumes, BROWN RICE, wheat germ and other foods high in vitamin B6 have a positive influence on eczema and other skin conditions. White rice, may cause eczema to flare up. Experiment and see if you can find a correlation between your diet and outbreaks of your eczema.

Rye: *(whole wheat)*

Eczema can be healed with the use of whole grains. RYE bread contains healing properties that helps eczema suffers. Gluten is a protein found mainly in wheat and to a lesser extent in RYE, this is usually seen in an Atopic individual & commonly associated with eczema. Just remember, there are many different products on the market, some containing drugs with dangerous side effects. An all natural diet will surely help you keep your eczema in check.

Spelt:

SPELT oil is said to be brilliant at healing eczema, SPELT is a predecessor of wheat & contains some gluten. Eczema sufferers have reported their symptoms seem to calm down after including spelt in their diet. If you have eczema use spelt flour instead of wheat. With eczema and most other skin disorders, the skin is being used as an organ and usually SPELT bread and other SPELT products are good alternatives to wheat.

Wheat: *for those of you who are not allergic to wheat*

WHEAT is available as a whole wheat grain (WHEAT berries), as flour, cracked and is often not the cause of eczema in adults. In some cases your eczema symptoms can be linked to a wheat allergy. Natural approaches to heal eczema and psoriasis, is to avoid grains containing gluten which include whole wheat. And SPELT is the perfect substitute for wheat.

Whole grain

There is no eczema natural cure, no magic pill or cream, but there are effective ways to keep it under control. The different types of whole grains work miracles in healing eczema. Eczema is a chronic, inflammatory skin disorder. Eat more fresh vegetables, whole grains, and essential fatty acids. Consume whole grains rather than white-flour products.

Part II

What Are The Causes Of Eczema?

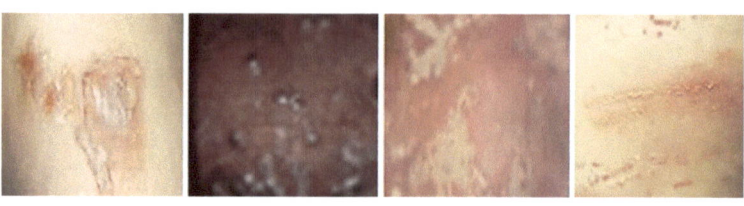

The causes of many types of eczema are quite apparent. One type of eczema, develops after frequent exposure to a mild irritant such as detergent or brief exposure to a strong irritant such as battery acid. Another type of allergic contact dermatitis develops when an allergen touches the skin and the person develops an allergic reaction. Common allergens include poison ivy and nickel. Many everyday and common objects contain nickel, which includes coins, jewellery, eyeglass frames and buttons. Believe it or not a nickel allergy is actually one of the most common causes of allergic contact dermatitis. Researchers believe that Atopic dermatitis develops when many factors are combined which include certain genes you inherit, overactive immune system and what dermatologists call a "barrier defect" which are "gaps in the skin" where water is lost too quickly. Although there is no way to cure eczema, there are steps you can take to avoid regular flare-ups. 1-Find Your Trigger Factor, 2-Eliminate Your Trigger Factors, 3-Avoid Too Much Direct Sunlight and 4-Keep the Skin Well Moisturized.

Causes Of Eczema

Atopic Dermatitis

Also known as "eczema," Atopic dermatitis is a chronic (non contagious) skin condition. It causes dry, itchy, irritated skin that can require daily skin care. Most people develop it before the age of 5 and usually get Atopic dermatitis from other family members. Approximately 10% to 20% of the world's population develops Atopic dermatitis. An estimated 65% develop Atopic dermatitis during their first year of life, and 90% develop the condition before age 5. While Atopic dermatitis often occur in many children by age 2, 50% usually continue to experience the signs and symptoms as hand eczema into adulthood.

Contact Dermatitis

Daily contact with everyday objects such as shampoo, jewellery, food and water is the cause of this very common type of eczema. When the contact irritated the skin, the eczema is called irritant contact dermatitis. Over time, the skin can become thick, red, scaly, darken and leathery after prolonged exposure to an allergen.

Dyshidrotic Dermatitis

This type of Dermatitis occurs when you get it only on the sides of your fingers, the palms of your hands and the soles of the feet causing a burning or itching sensation with blistering and rash.

Hand Dermatitis

Eczema which forms on the hands is not associated with any one specific type Dermatitis. Any type of eczema that develops on the hands can be classified as "hand dermatitis. Frequently job-related hand dermatitis often has different causes and can require special treatment.

Neurodermatitis

If you can imagine an itch so intense that no amount of scratching brings any type of relief what so ever, then you have an idea of what it feels like to have Neurodermatitis. Some factors could be insect bites and emotional stress.

Nummular Dermatitis

Developing on the skin after an injury, such as a burn, abrasion, or insect bite. One or many patches can develop that may last for weeks or even months.

Occupational Dermatitis

Occupational dermatitis is any type of eczema which developed at your place of work and a large number of people develop eczema on the job.

Seborrheic Dermatitis

Spreading to the face and beyond, this common type of eczema usually begins on the scalp as oily, waxy patches. Like most types of eczema, Seborrheic dermatitis tends to flare in cold as well as dry weather and sometimes produces widespread lesions.

These are just a few of the different types of Eczema which can make your life miserable. You might want to check the effects of Eczema Dermatitis out a little closer here and see what types of treatment might be available for your particular type Eczema. While Atopic dermatitis cannot be cured, most cases can be controlled with proper treatment. Treatment goals are to hydrate the skin, reduce inflammation, decrease the risk of infection, and get rid of the itchy rash. Despite many advertised claims, studies have not shown that the following food supplements can be helpful.

Evening primrose oil, Borage oil, Zinc, B6 (pyridoxine), and vitamin E.

Dairy Intolerance

This also includes Lactose intolerance which affects 3 out of every 4 people. It's all about allergic reactions and many people who suffer from eczema dermatitis and other problems have an allergic reaction to almost all dairy products. Because dairy sensitivity can be either Lactose Intolerance or milk protein allergy, you must be careful to distinguish between them. Lactose intolerance refer to a person's inability to digest Lactose, the sugar found in milk, and milk protein allergy refer to the body's allergic reaction to **Casein**. It is estimated that to some extent up to 75% of the world's population is Lactose intolerant. That is, three out of four people who have difficulty digesting lactose. And less than 3% are allergic to **Casein** (the protein found in milk). This is usually detected in babies but can remain undiagnosed till later in life. Dairy sensitivity is responsible for GI (gastro-intestinal) symptoms in millions of people and will become more noticeable now that thousands of processed foods contain dairy derivatives.

The symptoms of dairy intolerance include nausea, diarrhoea, bloating, flatulence and itchy skin conditions, GI (gastro-intestinal) and respiratory problems. Remember, Lactose intolerance should not be confused with Fructose intolerance, because many symptoms are the same. Lactose intolerance is known to increase markedly with age. To identify Dairy intolerance one has to be clinically tested which include the "Hydrogen" breath test and stool acidity tests. Dairy intolerance is all in the genes, generally you have a 75% chance of being Lactose intolerant, except if you are of Northern European ancestry the chance of Lactose intolerance is only 25%. Dairy sensitive people improve dramatically on a Dairy-free diet. Obviously the simplest strategy for managing Lactose intolerance is to go Dairy-free.

But before changing what you eat, and because Lactose intolerance is often confused with Fructose Intolerance you must positively identify your problem food. For Casein there needs to be more vigilance as Casein is now included in hundreds of processed foods. Actually there is no cure for dairy intolerance. But the symptoms will disappear when you remove dairy products from your diet. Once you have positively identified your problem food, you need a plan for long-term Dairy-free eating.

Yeast Sensitivity:
(Candida infections) is another allergic reaction that can make your eczema flare up and itch like crazy. Yeast infection is extremely common. Every one in three persons or 35% of people have yeast infections at any one given time. If this could be you, have your doctor check your symptoms. If you are sensitive to yeast get dramatic improvement on a yeast free diet. Yeast infection has a wide spectrum of symptoms of any food sensitivity; skin problems, gastro-intestinal problems, lethargy, headache, breathing difficulties, mood swings, you name it. Yeast infection is a disease that makes you feel "sick all over", and can be easily confused with other food intolerance like dairy and gluten intolerance. Although clinical testing is available, generally diagnosis is usually inconclusive.

The most useful indicator is the patient's history of yeast infection, such as ear or throat infections, jock itch, vaginal etc. Candida can also be notices through the appearance of stress or a compromised immune system, and anything that weakens the immune system can trigger a yeast infection. A combination of yeast-free diet and anti-fungal medication is the best way to treat yeast infections when they occur by inclusion or by accident in a wide variety of foods.

Gluten Sensitivity:

Gluten, and a small proportion to include Celiac and Wheat intolerance. Gluten intolerance is a broad term which includes all kinds of sensitivity, Gluten intolerant people will test positive to Celiac Disease test, and so are called Celiacs 0.5% of the population or 1 in 7. Gluten is a highly complex protein that occurs in four main grains. Wheat, rye, barley and oats. Gluten is present in all types of wheat grain such as whole grain wheat, bran, spelt, etc. and there are thousands of processed foods which contain Gluten. This also means that Gluten is present in all baked foods that are made from these grains: bread, pies, cake, breakfast cereals, porridge, cookies, pizza and pasta. Gluten is one of the most complex proteins consumed by man and is difficult for the human digestive system to break down. Some Gluten intolerance is identified in childhood and manifests itself with headaches, mouth ulcers, weight gain or loss, poor immunity to disease and skin problems like dermatitis and eczema. So in your quest for an eczema free life make sure that you test for Gluten intolerance with your doctor, avoid these types of foods and improve your eczema dramatically within weeks on a Gluten-free diet.

Fructose or Sugar sensitivity:

Hereditary Fructose Intolerance is quite rare (less than one in 10,000). It is inherited and lasts for life. Fructose is found in processed foods like soft drinks and confectionery. Sugar cravings are strongly associated with Fructose sensitivity, and the symptoms of Fructose sensitivity are very similar to Lactose Intolerance so they can be misdiagnosed. Long term effects are poor and sensitive skin, nails and hair; general ill health and even osteoporosis. Treatment of Fructose Intolerance (HFI) is a very strict Fructose-free diet with NO FRUIT or fruit juice for life. Consider the high level of sugars we ingest; soft drinks, confectionery, desserts and thousands of processed foods and pharmaceuticals. Fructose sensitive people improve dramatically on a low-sugar Fructose-free Diet. It is estimated that around 3% of children and about 1% of adults have some kind of Food Allergy. Often the allergens are in shellfish, eggs, milk, nuts, soy, wheat, corn, and fish. They can also be found in food additives like colours and preservatives. Food allergy symptoms are typically SUDDEN ONSET AND SEVERE. There can be ear, nose, throat and respiratory problems like nasal congestion and asthma. Skin problems like dermatitis, eczema, hives or rashes and gastro-intestinal disorders like nausea and vomiting. Food allergies are an autoimmune response caused by the body 'misreading' a food protein as an enemy or toxic substance. Because they are fairly dramatic, allergic responses are usually easily identified with blood tests or "patch testing". Now you might ask-how did I get a Food Allergy? Often when a child is allergic, there are family members with allergies or a tendency for allergies to be passed on. Others develop allergies with no apparent genetic background. Treatment is generally one of three approaches: largely it involves avoidance of the allergen whenever possible, *treatment and management* of symptoms, or *auto-immune therapy* - injections of extracts of the allergen to try and de-sensitise the individual.

You can depend 100% on an improved natural diet as the only remedy for reversing eczema. Whole or organic food supplements can be attributed to a large percent to the success rate in reversing many people's eczema after using these wild-crafted, organic natural whole food supplements for their eczema treatment. Whole food supplements are far superior in quality and effectiveness for reversing eczema because they are produced in their natural and complex configuration. A natural eczema treatment is to supplement your body with nutrient rich foods. The "Nutritional Medicine" approach includes principles that are of great benefit to the treatment of eczema. Therefore, when choosing a diet to help control your eczema dermatitis skin, there are several factors you needs to consider in order to reduce flare ups, all the while ensuring that you get the nutrients that you need to be a healthy and thriving individual.

Organic Foodstuffs:
Raw foods like fruits, vegetables, and sprouts are known to have a marked effect on the B cells function. These cells are the lymphocytes which play a big role in the humoral immune response, functioning mainly to make antibodies fight against antigens. So in short, these raw foods boost the production of lymphocytes in order to enhance the body's resistance to ill health. By taking in raw foods, the body is supplied with good quantities of vitamins A, C, E, B, and zinc. This then will result in a powerful immune system, protecting the body from diseases like eczema and maintaining smooth and healthier skin. These are the basic steps that my brother took to help control his intestinal hygiene and his complete diet.

But I would suggest that before you start your program to consult your doctor or try and find a nutrition coach to help you get through the program. The above statements have not been evaluated by the Food and Drug

Administration. These products are not intended to
diagnose, treat, cure or prevent any disease. I hope that
this small booklet will be of some help to you in your
struggle against eczema troubled skin. These are only a
few of the many herbs that can be beneficial in the fight
against acne, eczema and other types of skin diseases.

Part III

Special Tasty Homeopathic Natural Grain Eczema Curing Salads

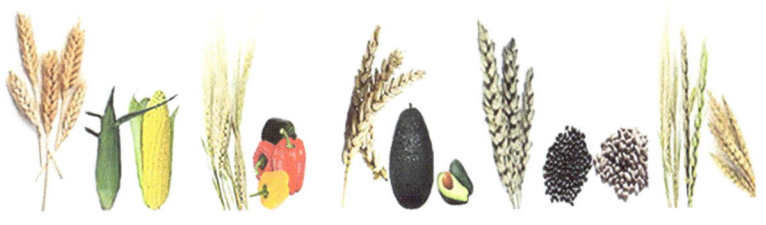

Rich in omega3 fatty acids, not only do they taste GREAT, these salads are also rich in vitamins and nutrients and they can also help you in your fight against eczema and troubled skin. If you are on a special diet try some of these eczema-salads, you will love them, they are extremely healthy, and provides you with eczema healing nutrients that you just don't get with normal salads or meals. If you are on a wheat free diet for instance, my Green (whole grain) SPELT (*which is an ancient form of wheat*) salad would be just what the doctor ordered. These are the exact same salads that my brother used and consumed to help fight off his eczema, and you can do the same. And even if you are a Vegan or your skin is eczema free I'm sure that you will enjoy these natural whole grain homeopathic herbal salads. These are the original grain receipts so if you are allergic to any of the ingredients you should try and substitute them with another grain. Even though some of these salads are made with yogurt and cheese, and some of you may be lactos intolerant, never the less these wonder salads are rich in nutrients and vitamins, and high in fatty acids. In order for these to taste as they should please try and stick with the order in which they are presented to you, this is important… Depending on the type of eczema that you have, some of the ingredients may cause unwanted effects. In this case substitute for instance "wheat" with "spelt" if you have an intolerance to wheat. Enjoy your salads and I am sure that they will be effective in your fight against eczema troubled skin.

INGREDIENTS FOR SALADS

- BARLEY
- BAY LEAVES
- BUCK WHEAT
- CEYANNE PEPPER
- CLOVES
- CRÈME FRAICH
- CAN CORN
- CHEESE
- CURRY
- FENNEL
- GARLIC
- GARLIC POWDER
- GREEN OLIVES
- HERBAL VINEGAR
- HOT MUSTARD
- HOT PAPRIKA
- HORSERADISH
- YOGURT
- LENON JUICE
- MILLET
- NATURAL RICE
- NUT MEG
- OATMEAL FLAKES
- RED BENS
- SAMBOL OELEK

- SOUR CREAM
- SOUR PICKLES
- SPELT
- THICK APPLE JUICE
- TABASCO SAUC
- TOMATOES
- WHOLE GRAIN KERNELS
- TOMATOES
- WHOLE GRAIN KERNELS
- WHITE BEANS
- WINE VINEGAR
- WHITE PEPPER
- WHOLE WHEAT GRAIN
- WHOLE RYE GRAIN

COOKING INSTRUCTIONS FOR WHOLE GRAIN

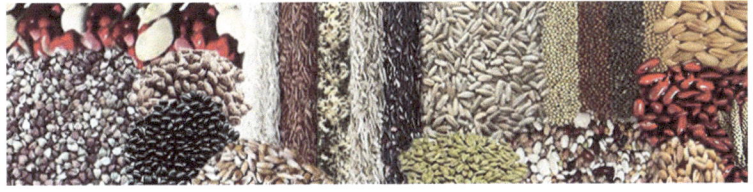

GREEN grain - or SPELT

Green corn is made from *SPELT* which is a very ancient type of wheat that is harvested while it is still green, so that you can kiln-dry them. This process causes them to ripen more and help start and supports the digestive process in humans. *SPELT* is almost always found in herbal kitchens. This medieval wheat grain has less gluten than traditional wheat, therefore it is a good substitute if you are sensitive to wheat and wheat products. For the preparation of dishes made of whole grain, one can use either bruised grain, whole meal grain or prepare them whole. In this case it is important to prepare the grain so that it's for humans easy to digest. After you have washed the grain well under running water (*only buckwheat has to be washed in hot water*) soak the grain in cold water 3-10 hours. You should not exceed this time period because after ten hours the grain will start to sprout. For buckwheat, millet, rice, bruised grain or whole meal grain, it is not necessary to soak, and it does shortens the cooking time.

Using the same water that you soaked the grain in, bring to a boil, and then let simmer at the lowest setting for 20-50 minutes in a closed pot with top to gar. After cooking time is over, the burner is out, let pot sit on burner for a while to continue to soak, or in a thermos to expand and let soak for some time. You should test the grain to make sure that it doesn't get too soft. A rule of thumb: as far as the amount of water needed to soak grain, use twice as much water as grain, 1-cup grain = 2 cups water. Sometimes during the soaking process you may want to add a little more water. Do not use any salt until the soaking process is almost complete, i.e. until the grain has absorbed most of the liquid. You get a spicy taste when you gar the grain in vegetable bullion; this way you can use the grain for salads or other dishes that you wish to make, or use them as condiments. In this case you should use a little oil or herbal seasoning. You decorate the finished grain with green herbs and mix with coloured veggies or bake with dark yellow cheese.

Special Ingredients:

MAPLE SYRUP:

Use thin flowing maple syrup which is taken from young maple trees, it's less sweeter than honey.

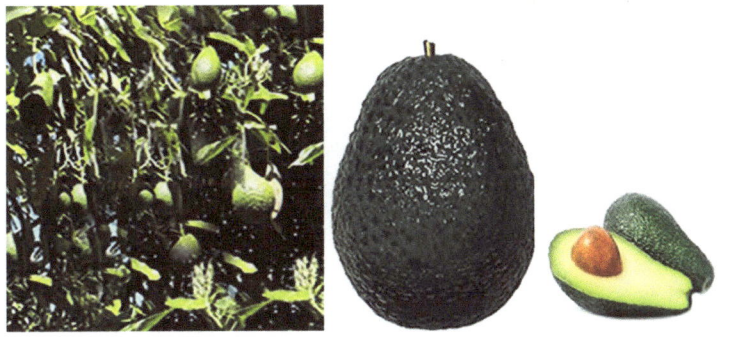

AVOCADO DIP

Avocado will help to eliminate your Eczema if included in your diet... AVOCADO carrier oil is quite beneficial in treating skin diseases, it is extremely beneficial in treating skin disorders such as Eczema and Psoriasis. Skin problems, especially Eczema and psoriasis, respond to its high content of vitamins A and E. Eat lots of AVOCADOS and other foods high in EFAs (essential fatty acids) not only will your Eczema be under control you will feel great all the time

INGREDIENTS:
1- LARGR RIP AVOCADO
2 TS LEMON JUICE
1 PRESSED GARLIC TOOTH
SALT
CEYANNE PEPPER
2 TBS MAYONNAISE
1-CUP SOUR CREAM (store bought)

PREPARATION:
Cut avocado in half, take out seed and spoon out the meat of the fruit and mash fine with a fork. Add lemon juice, garlic, cayenne pepper, mayonnaise and sour cream -mix well season to taste with salt.

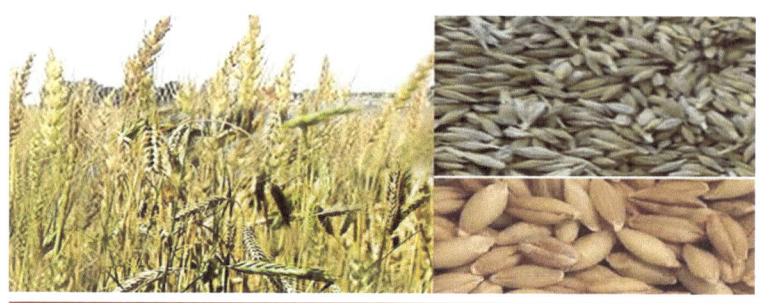

BARLEY-SALAD - for 10 Servings

BARLEY grass may be used to alleviate ECZEMA. The high chlorophyll content in BARLEY grass gives it strong cleansing properties and gets rid of toxins in the body. Many people are allergic to Barley, and if you are, try an alternative grain for this salad. BARLEY Grass (12 grams of BARLEY Grass powder administered in 3 x 4 gram dosages per day) may alleviate ECZEMA (in up to 75% of patients).

INGREDIENTS:
500g (17,6oz) BARLEY GRAIN
1 PACKAGE FROZEN PEAS
1-CAN SWEET YELLOW CORN WITHOUT JUICE
1-RED FINELY CUBED PAPRIKA
1- YELLOW (or GREEN) FINELY CUBED PAPRIKA
2-CUBED MEAT TOMATOES
200g (7,1oz) YOUNG GAUDA CHEESE CUBED
200g (7,1oz) DUTCH EMMENTALER CHEESE CUBED
6-8 CUBED SAUER PICKLES

MARINADE:
8-TBS WHITE WINE VINEGAR
16-TBS OIL+ APP. ½ TS SALT
1-TS GARLIC POWDER
APP. 1-TS FRESH GROUND BLACK PEPPPER

LOTS OF CUT SEASONAL HERBS (PARCLEY, DILL ETC.) OR
1 PACK DEEP FROZEN SEASONAL HERBS: all in all you
need app. 4-8 different types of herbs.

PREPARATION:

Bring Barley to a boil in about 1 ½ litres app. 2 pints of
water, then let simmer on lowest setting for app 35 min. and
make sure that they don't get too soft. Soak herbs and
seasoning, i.e. pepper salt and garlic powder together in the
vinegar for a short while. After, that mix with the oil, then
the veggies and cheese and mix in the marinade. Mix good
and let set for a while…yummy!

Variation:

Change this receipt into a noodle salad by substituting
500g (17,6oz) noodles for the barley.

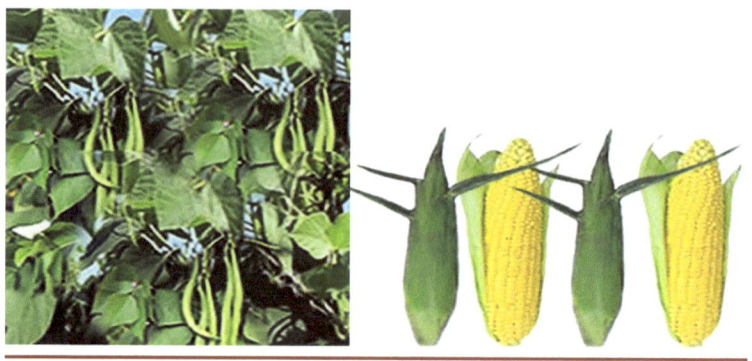

BEAN AND CORN-SALAD - for 8 Servings

Kidney bean, common bean, green bean, navy bean, string bean, wax bean. Prolonged use of the decoction made from beans is recommended for difficult cases of acne. Bean meal can be applied directly to the skin for moist eczema, eruptions and itching. Even though some people have an intolerance to corn, others don't. Corn is a common food that may act as triggers to your eczema eruptions. Eating organic corn may help to get rid of this problem and has helped control eczema in many cases. If you are allergic to corn try substituting it with another grain such as Bulgar.

INGREDIENTS
2- CUPS COOKED WHITE BEANS
2- =   =   RED BEANS
2- =   =   CAN CORN
2- =   =   LARGE TOMATOES (CUT IN FINE STRIPES)
1- CUCUMBER
SALT, PEPPER
½ TS-SUGAR
1-PRESSED GARLIC TOOTH
150G (5,2oz) GRATED CHEESE

FOR THE SAUCE:

SALT, PEPPER
PINCH OF PAPRIKA
¼ TS-SUGAR
¼ CUP LEMON JUICE OR WHITE WINE VINEGAR
¾ CUP OLIVE OIL
1 PRESSED GARLIC TOOTH
1TBS CHOPPED ONIONS

TO DECORATE:

LETTUCE AND 150g (5,2oz) CUBED CHEESE

PREPARATION:

Put the above ingredients in a large bowl and mix good together…but before, mix the herbs and garlic with cheese and sit in fridge for 2 hours. Mix the ingredients for the sauce 30 minutes before serving. Place the mixture (beans, corn, tomatoes etc.) on the lettuce (you will need a large plate) and pour the sauce over the mixture, garnish with cheese. Presto!

Eczema Curing Salads

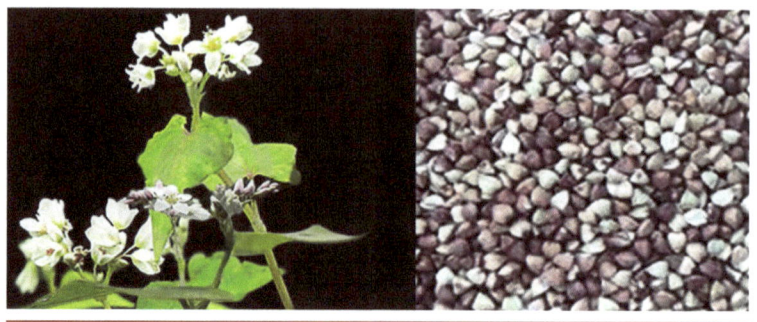

BUCKWHEAT-SALAD- for 4-6 Servings

BUCKWHEAT is the seed of the herbaceous plant *Fagopyrum esculentum Moench* and has been used as a homeopathic medicine in cases of severe itching and ECZEMA. BUCKWHEAT tea is used to cure circulatory problems. It is also used in the treatment of chilblain, retinitis and liver disorders.

INGREDIENTS:
1-CUP BUCKWHEAT
1-EGG
2- CUPS BOILING WATER
1-2 TSB POWERED VEGETABLE BULLION (1-2 Cubes)
1-SMALL GREEN PAPRIKA CUBED
3-TOMATOES
150g-(5,2oz) 200g (7,1oz) FRESH CUCUMBER
1-SMALL CHOPPED ONION
1-SMALL OR ½ FENNEL CHOPPED FINE
100g (3,5oz) CUBED EMMENTALER CHEESE
CHOPPED FENNEL LEAVES OR PARSLEY

MARINADE:
3-4 TBS CORN OR OLIVE OIL
2-3 TBS HERBAL VINEGAR
PEPPER, SALT, SUGAR

PREPARATION:

Wash buckwheat in hot water and place in a large pot, stir in the egg. Continue stirring by normal heat until the buckwheat kernels (grain) begin to separate and become drier. Pour in the 2 cups of boiling water, add the bullion and stir good. Reduce heat to the lowest level, place lid on pot and let cook 20-30 minutes long. The kernels should not be too soft. After cooking cool buckwheat. Mix the cold buckwheat with the rest of the vegetables, then add the cheese and marinade, season to taste.

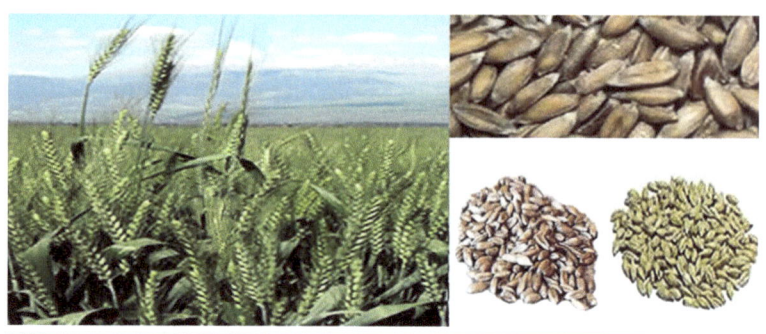

COLORFUL GREEN GRAIN/ Spelt/ SALAD- for 4-6 servings

SPELT oil is said to be brilliant at healing Eczema, SPELT is the predecessor of wheat & contains some gluten. Eczema sufferers have reported their symptoms seem to calm down after including spelt in their diet. With Eczema and most other skin disorders, the skin is being used as an organ and usually SPELT bread and other SPELT products are good alternatives to wheat.

INGREDIENTS:
250g (8,9oz) SPELT
½ LITER (APP. 1 PINT) STRONG VEGETABLE BULLION
1 LARGE RED + 1 YELLOW PAPRIKA
½ BUNDLE SPRING ONIONS
1-CAN CORN OR OTHER CAN VEGGIES
OIL, VINEGAR, SALT, PEPPER or OIL LEMON, SALT AND PEPPER
PINCH OF SUGAR
GARLIC (TO TASTE)
4-8 DIFFERENT TYPES FRESH (or frozen) CUT GARDEN HERBS

PREPARATION:
Soak the green grain and cook in vegetable stock until gar, (see instructions for cooking grain) remove kernels from pot and place in refrigerator. Cut spring onions, and paprika in thin stripes and mix with spelt and corn. Then

make a marinade with the rest of the ingredients, pour over salad and mix well- let stand for a while-season to taste and add 4-6 different types of fresh or fresh frozen garden herbs.

Tip:
You can influence the taste greatly with more salt and lemon juice.

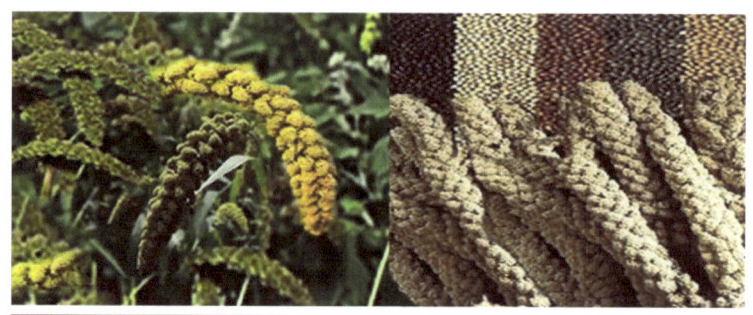

MILLET-SALAD for 4-6 Servings

Atopic eczematous dermatitis is one of the most common forms of ECZEMA, MILLET is far removed from the family of grains to which wheat belongs to. A gluten free diet is often very beneficial in treating ECZEMA and psoriasis. Add brown rice and MILLET to your diet and be sure to include plenty of fibber. The green leaves of finger MILLET are valuable in chronic ECZEMA. The fresh juice of these leaves should be applied over the affected area in the treatment.

INGREDIENTS:
20g APP. (1-OZ) PLANT MARGARINE
1-SMALL CUT ONION
150g (5,2oz) MILLET
APP. 400ml (14oz) STRONG VEGETABLE BROTH OR
BULLION
150g CUBED CARROTS
1-BAY LEAF
150g COOKED PEAS
2-CUBED HERB PICKLES (NOT SAUER)
4-TBS OIL
JUICE FROM 1 LEMON
MUSTARD
THICK APPLE JUICE
SALT, PEPPER and a PINCE OF GARLIC POWDER

PREPARATION:

Wash millet-cook onions in margarine until glassy- add millet and let simmer for a few minutes, then add the broth with bay leaf and let simmer on low flame app. 20 minutes in a pot with lid on it. Remove the bay leaf and let cool. Mix together with the carrots, peas and pickles. Make a sauce with the rest of the ingredients (add more water if need be) and mix with millet mixture. Let stand to soak in the ingredients, decorate with fresh parsley. This is an unforgettable taste!!!

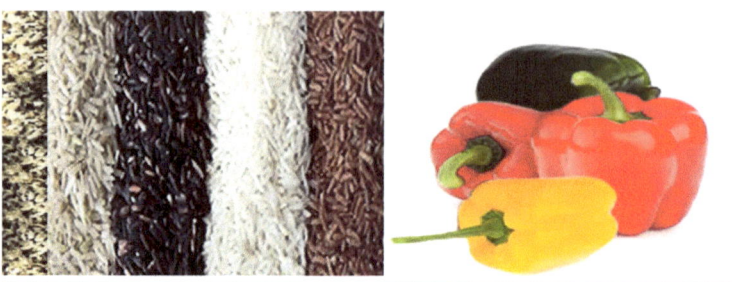

PAPRICA RICE-SALAT for 8 servings

In some cases paprika is used for Atopic dermatitis and ECZEMA treatment, but to my knowledge many eczema suffers are allergic to it. If this is not the case for you, this salad will bring you much joy and satisfaction. Eating plenty of legumes, BROWN RICE, wheat germ and other foods high in vitamin B6 have a positive influence on ECZEMA and other skin conditions. White rice may cause ECZEMA to flare up. Test this salad first and see if it causes your eczema to flare up, if so change to brown rice.

INGREDIENTS:
400g (14oz) WHOLE NATURAL LONG CORN RICE-COOK
ADENTE´
2-RED PAPRICA-FINE CUBED
2-GREEN PAPRIKA FINE CUBED
ADD FRESH MUSHROOMS AND CUBED CHEESE
ACCORDING TO TASTE

MARINADE:
1 MEDIUM SIZE ONION
50g (1,7oz) PARCLEY CHOPPED FINE
4 TBS MAYONNAISE OR MIRACLE WHIP
1-2 TBS LEMON JUICE
1 PRESSED GARLIC TOOTH

½ TS SAMBOL OELEK
1-TS THYME, SALT AND FRESH GROUND NUTMEG

PREPARATION:
Mix the marinade well, then mix with the ingredients mentioned above. Let stand app. 1 hour. Decorate with sliced hard boiled eggs and green olives. Also good as cold buffet. A good substitute for rice would be Bulgar.

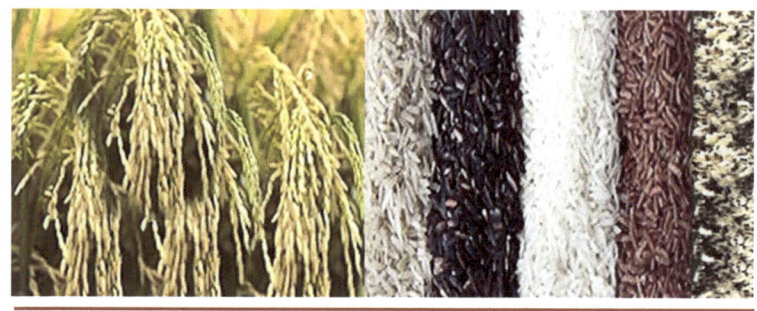

ORIENTAL RICE-SALAD for 4-6 servings

Eating plenty of legumes, BROWN RICE, wheat germ and other foods high in vitamin B6 have a positive influence on ECZEMA and other skin conditions. White rice, may cause ECZEMA to flare up. Experiment and see if you can find a correlation between your diet and outbreaks of your eczema.

INGREDIENTS:
150g (5,2oz) NATURAL OR LONG GRAIN RICE, TRY BASMATI
250g (8,9oz) COOKED GREEN BEANS
4-CUBED TOMAOES
2-CUBED RED PAPRIKE

MARINADE:
1-GARLIC TOOTH
1 ½ TS HOT MUSTAD
6-TBS OLIVE OIL
2-TBS HERBAL VINEGAR
3-DASHES OF TOBASCO SAUCE
WHITE PEPPER
CURRY
PINCE OF SUGAR

PREPARATION:

Cook rice, let cool and mix with veggies. For the marinade mash the garlic with salt, and mix well with mustard. Pour over the salad, mix well and let sit in refrigerator for 30 minutes to soak in the ingredients. Decorate with sliced hard boiled eggs and tomatoes. Right here I would like to say that in cases such as beans, carrots, peas etc. and if you do not want to use can food, you can use fresh out of the garden or produce store vegetables. First, steam cook them in a vegetable bullion for 15-20 min depending on the vegetable making sure that they are not over cooked. Let cool and then mix together with the rest of the ingredients. I prefer to use fresh vegetables because I can make sure that most of the eczema fighting and other vital nutrients remain in the vegetable.

Even if you are not suffering from eczema or some other type of chronic skin disease, once you eat these salads you will ***never*** ***ever*** give them up…

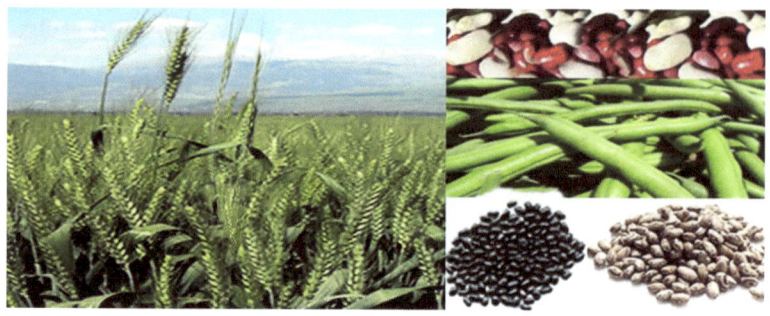

SPELT AND BEAN SALAD for 6-8 Servings

If you have eczema, use spelt flour instead of wheat. With ECZEMA and most other skin disorders, the skin is being used as an organ and usually SPELT bread and other SPELT products are good alternatives to wheat. Prolonged use of the decoction made from beans is recommended for difficult cases of acne and eczema. Bean meal can be applied directly to the skin for moist eczema, eruptions and itching.

INGREDIENTS:

300g (10,5oz) COOKED SPELT OR 150g (5,2oz) UNCOOKED
400g (14oz) COOKED GREEN BEANS
200g (7,1oz) CUBED APPENZELLER CHEESE
1-ONION
2-TOMATOES
3 TBS OIL
2-3 TBS VINEGAR
Pepper, Salt, a Pinch of sugar add a little garlic if you like,
Parsley, Basel and Savoury chopped well.

PREPARATION:

Soak the grain and cook as directed. Let cool and mix with beans, onions, tomatoes and cheese. With the rest of the ingredients make a sauce, pour over salad and let stand a few minutes to soak up the ingredients, check seasoning. Mmmm, Very Tasty…

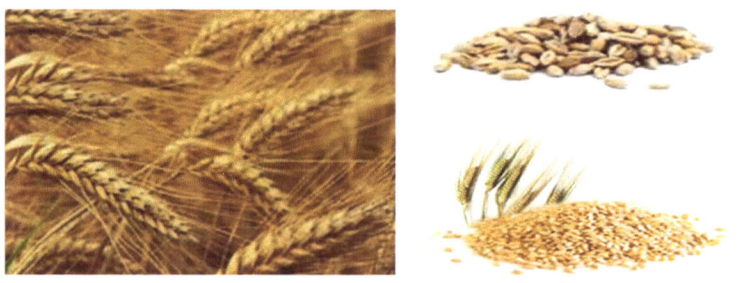

SPICY WHEAT SALAD for 5-6 Servings

WHEAT is available as a WHOLE grain (WHEAT berries), as flour, cracked, and is often not the cause of ECZEMA in adults. In some cases your ECZEMA symptoms can be linked to a WHEAT allergy. Natural approaches to heal ECZEMA and psoriasis, is to avoid grains containing gluten, which include WHOLE WHEAT, and SPELT is the perfect substitute for wheat.

INGREDIENTS:
250g (8,9oz) WHOLE WHEAT KERNELS
APP. 200g (7,1oz) RED BEETS
APP. 200g (7,1oz) COOKED CELERY
2-3 PICKLES
1 CUP CUT PINEAPPLE
100g (3,5oz) CHOPPED NUTS (YOUR CHOICE)
4-TBS OIL
3-TBS VINEGAR
3-TBS SOUR CREAM OR CRÈME FRAICH
1-TS HERBAL SALT
1-PINCE CAYENNE PEPPER
1-TBS CAPERS
PINEAPPLE JUICE

PREPARATION:

Soak the kernels according to instructions and cook until soft-but not too soft. Cut red beets, pickles and celery in small cubes or stripes and mix everything together with the pineapples and nuts. With the rest of the ingredients make a sauce, pour over the salad and mix well. Test for seasoning and let stand and marinade until serving. If you use pickled beets or celery use less vinegar.

Variation:

For a different taste use pineapple, nuts, 1 cubed apple and 1 cubed medium size onion.

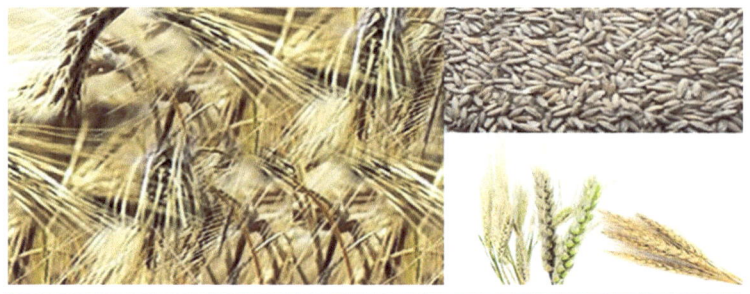

WHOLE GRAIN RYE SALAD - for 5-6 Servings

Eczema healed with the use of whole grains. RYE bread contains healing power that helps ECZEMA suffers. Gluten is a protein found mainly in wheat and to a lesser extent in RYE, this is usually seen in an Atopic individual & commonly associated with ECZEMA.

INGREDIENTS:
250g (8,9oz) WHOLE GRAIN RYE KERNELS
2-3- CLOVES (NELKEN)
1-2- BAY LEAVES
PEPER OR CORN PEPPER
SALT
1-JAR RED BEETS 400g (14oz) TO 500g (17,6oz)
2-LARGE SOUR APPLES

MARINADE:
½ TS MUSTARD, FRUIT VINEGAR, OR LEMON JUICE
A LITTLE JUICE FROM THE BEETS
APP. 1-TL SUNFLOWER, OR THISTLE OIL
1-TBS HORSERADISH
SALT- PEPPER OR CAYENNE PEPPER - LITTLE SUGAR
½ PLASTIC CUP CRÈME FRAICH, OR EQUAL AMOUNTS OF
MIRACLE WHIP OR MAYONNAISE
½ cup NATURAL YOGURT

Soak the Rye kernels. Cook cloves, bay leaves, pepper, and salt in water or with veggie bullion (1-2 ½) until they are soft. Remove from stove, and let cool. Cut apples and beets in cubes or slices and mix with the rye grain (When you make the marinade use all of the ingredients except the yogurt and mayonnaise). Mix together and let stand until serving. Before serving add the yogurt and mayonnaise and mix well. If needed, season to taste with a bit more vinegar, pepper and brown sugar.

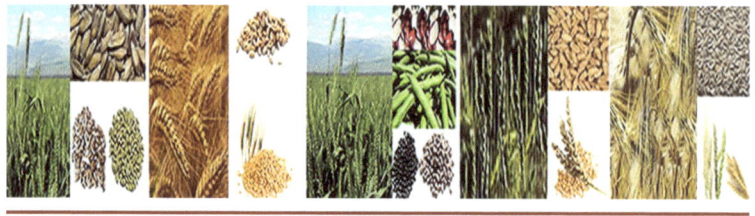

WHOLE GRAIN SALAD for 4-6 Servings

There is no ECZEMA natural cure, no magic pill or cream, but there are effective ways to keep it under control. The different types of all natural "Whole Grains" work miracles in healing ECZEMA and Psoriasis skin. ECZEMA is a chronic, inflammatory skin disorder. Eat more fresh vegetables, WHOLE GRAINS, and essential fatty acids.

INGREDIENTS:
300g (10,5oz) OF YOUR FAVOURITE COOKED WHOLE GRAIN KERNELS
PEAS, BEANS, PAPRIKA, CARROTS, CORN, SPRING ONIONS, CUCUMBER etc.
APP. 150g (5,2oz) TOMATOES CUBED FINE

MARINADE:
1-CUP SOUR CREAM
1-CUP YOGURT
1-TBS MUSTARD
HERBAL VINEGAR, SALT IF NEEDED, HORSERADISH
2-HARD COOKED EGGS CUBED
LOTS OF FRESH HERBS NOT TOO FINELY CHOPPED

PREPARATION:
Cook grain according to instructions and let cool. Mix the marinade and the veggies together. Let stand for a while-if need be add more salt and decorate. Guten Appetite!

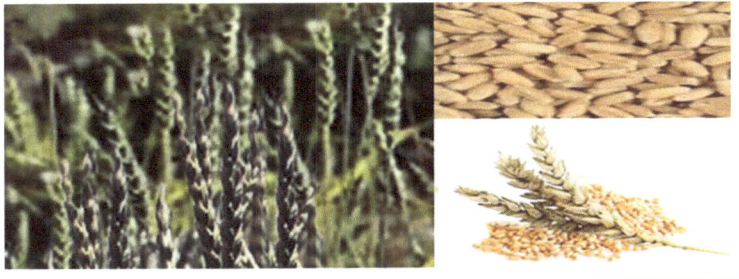

WHEAT SALAD for 4-6 Servings

WHEAT is available as a WHOLE grain, as flour, cracked, and is often not the cause of ECZEMA in most adults. In some cases your ECZEMA symptoms can be linked to a WHEAT allergy. The best way to approach and heal your ECZEMA and psoriasis, is to avoid foods containing gluten, which include WHOLE WHEAT, and SPELT is the perfect substitute for wheat.

INGREDIENTS:
250g (8,9oz) WHEAT GRAIN KERNELS
2 ½ CUP YOGURT
¼ CUP OIL
1-TS SALT
1-TS HOT PAPRIKA POWDER
½ TS CURRY
2-LARGE SWEETAPPLES
3-MEDIUM SIZE PICKLES
1-MEDIUM SIZE ONION
4-6 TBS MAYONNAISE OR MIRACLE WHIP
3-TBS OATMEAL FLAKES

PREPARATION:
Soak wheat and let cook until gar. Chop the onions and cut the apple and pickles in fine cubes. With the rest of the ingredients make a sauce and mix everything together.

Finally add the cooled wheat kernels and let stand 3-4 hours before serving. Yummy yum yum!!

Tip:
I like yogurt that I make myself. If you can make your own yogurt it would give the salad an even greater taste.

About the ingredients

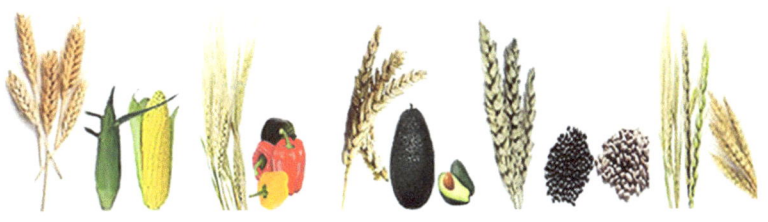

As we all know different foods cause different types of eczema to flare up, and some of the ingredients used in these salads, may cause your eczema to flare up as well. and if this is the case try and substitute the ingredient(s) that is causing the flare up. If you have a Lactos intolerance try soy products.

Home remedies for eczema are used as alternatives for prescription medications and some over-the-counter products. Many sufferers opt for home remedies because they are safer. There are fewer risks and side effects. Your goal is to seek treatment, not have other medical issues and complications to deal with as well. When using home remedies to treat eczema, you may need to purchase a few more supplies, but they are pretty affordable when compared to getting and using prescription medications. Moreover, you may already have what you need inside your home. In that case, no additional money is needed to seek relief. Not only does avoiding the doctor save you money, but it also eliminates a major hassle. If you work outside of the home or you are a parent, you must arrange time between work and childcare. Don't loose money or time with your kids, because home remedies enable you to treat your eczema from home and with ease. If you suffer from eczema, you want and need to seek relief. You may opt for expensive over-the-counter products or try other prescriptions recommended by your doctor.

These may work, but don't discount natural ways to fight off eczema. Luckily, there are many natural remedies that have proven effective for treating eczema and when it comes to treating and managing the disease, sufferers have many choices. You may have heard that home remedies work, but do they? Although our bodies are all different, they have proven effective for millions of people. That is just one of many reasons why natural home remedies are recommended for the treatment of eczema. Although results are not guaranteed, many eczema patients have used home remedies to seek relief from the constant outbreak of itchy, irritated skin.

Home remedies for eczema are used as alternatives for prescription medications and some over the counter products. Many sufferers opt for home remedies because they are safer. If you are interested in more information about home remedies please stay tuned for my up coming book on eczema irritated skin disorders called "Eczema Herbal Treatments".

DISCLAIMER

THE ABOVE STATEMENTS HAVE NOT BEEN EVALUATED BY THE FOOD AND DRUG ADMINISTRATION. THESE PRODUCTS ARE NOT INTENDED TO DIAGNOSE, TREAT, CURE OR PREVENT ANY DISEASE.

These pages are presented solely as a source of INFORMATION and ENTERTAINMENT and to provide stern warnings against use where appropriate. No claims are made for the efficacy of any herb or for any historical herbal treatment. In no way can the information provided here take the place of the standard, legal, medical practice of any country.

you choose to do with this information. Use your own judgment. Any perceived slight of specific people or organizations, and any resemblance to characters living, dead or otherwise, real or fictitious, is purely unintentional. In practical advice books, like anything else in life there are no guarantees of income made. Readers are cautioned to reply on their own judgment about their individual circumstances to act accordingly. You are encouraged to print this book for easy reading. Use this information at your own risk.

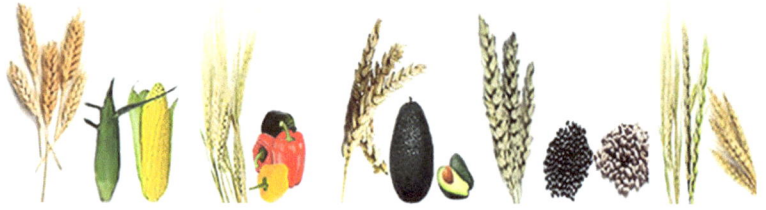

Eczema And The Food We Eat

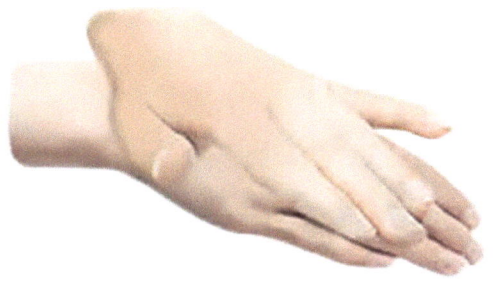

CreateSpace Direct
Bookstore and Online Retailer
Web: http://www.eczemaherbalcures.com

ISBN-13: 978-1499592825
ISBN-10: 1499592825
Title ID: 4796220

10 9 8 7 6 5 4 3

First Edition, first printing: May 2014
Printed in the United States Of America

www.ingramcontent.com/pod-product-compliance
Lightning Source LLC
Chambersburg PA
CBHW050822290526
45792CB00001B/217